I0105447

Parliaments, politics and HIV/AIDS

Canadian
International
Development
Agency

Agence
canadienne de
développement
international

CanadaFund
for Africa

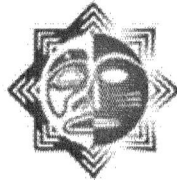

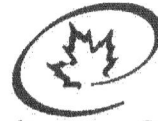

Parliamentary Centre
le Centre parlementaire

Canada

idasa

This report is a synthesis report from a comparative study in Botswana, Ghana, Kenya, Mozambique and South Africa on the effective use of parliamentary oversight in respect of the national responses to HIV/AIDS. The project was made possible by the Canadian Parliamentary Centre via the Africa-Canada Parliamentary Strengthening Programme funded by the Canadian International Development Agency through the Canada Fund for Africa, and coordinated and implemented by the Governance and AIDS Programme of Idasa (Idasa-GAP)

Published by Idasa, 6 Spin Street, Cape Town
© Governance and AIDS Programme, Idasa, 2006
First published 2006

ISBN 1-920118-22-5
ISBN-13: 978-1-920118-22-8

Editing, design and production by Idasa Publishing
Cover design by Magenta Media

All rights reserved. No part of this publication may be reproduced or transmitted, in any form or by any means, without prior permission from the publisher.

PARLIAMENTS, POLITICS AND HIV/AIDS

A comparative study of five African countries

Prepared by Mary Caesar-Katsenga and Marietjie Myburg

2006

IDASA's Governance and AIDS Programme

Idasa is an independent public interest organisation committed to promoting sustainable democracy in South Africa and elsewhere by building democratic institutions, educating citizens and advocating social justice.

The Governance and AIDS Programme conducts innovative research to provide evidence of the impact of HIV/AIDS on governance and to raise wider awareness through strategic and general dissemination of findings

GAP staff:

Kondwani Chirambo, programme manager
Vasanthie Naicker, administrator
Marietjie Myburg, regional co-ordinator (communication)
Mary Caesar-Katsenga, research facilitator
Josina Machel, co-ordinator, capacity building
Nhlanhla Ndlovu, manager, AIDS Budget Unit
Rabelani Daswa, researcher/ trainer, AIDS Budget Unit
Nobuntu Mbebetho, research assistant, AIDS Budget Unit

Acknowledgements

This research project was a collaboration between the Canadian Parliamentary Centre (PC) and Idasa's Governance and AIDS Programme (Idasa-GAP). We would like to thank the Canadian PC for their programmatic input and financial support. In particular, we thank Ms Christine Ivory, regional co-ordinator, Parliamentary Support Programme, Mr Steven Langdon, director of the Africa-Canada Parliamentary Support Programme and Ms Anna Miller, who was a staff member of the PC when the project started.

This synthesis report was compiled from research papers prepared by the five participating countries: Botswana, Ghana, Kenya, Mozambique and South Africa. Idasa-GAP thanks the institutions, the researchers and the research assistants for their work:

- Botswana: The Southern African Centre for Policy Development and Dialogue, research coordinator, Dr Gloria Somolekae.
- Ghana: The Centre for Democratic Development (CDD), research coordinator, Mr Franklin Odoro.
- Kenya: Department of Economics, University of Nairobi and the Institute of Policy Analysis and Research (IPAR), research coordinator, Dr Urbanus Kioko.
- Mozambique: Ms Josina Machel, independent research consultant based in Maputo (now with Idasa-GAP).
- South Africa: Idasa, research coordinators, Mr Nhlanhla Ndlovu (AIDS Budget Unit) and Ms Mary Caesar-Katsenga (Idasa-GAP).

We are grateful for the contributions of a number of interns who were based at Idasa's Pretoria office. In particular Mr Ryan Schwartz of Stanford University for literature review, editing, comments on the country reports and for commenting on previous versions of the synthesis report.

All the researchers thank Members of Parliament and resource persons in the five countries for their participation in the project.

Kondwani Chirambo, programme manager
Mary Caesar-Katsenga, research facilitator

Contents

Page

Tables

Page

Foreword

The HIV/AIDS pandemic is increasingly being acknowledged as a growing governance challenge. As HIV/AIDS hurts economic and social growth by draining poor nations of their children, workers and leaders, it puts pressure on political systems and can challenge democracy.

Strong leadership is required to effectively combat the pandemic. The greatest achievements in preventing the spread of the disease and alleviating the impact of AIDS has been found in countries where the political leadership has demonstrated strong political will and firm commitment to acknowledge and respond to the crisis openly and as a national priority.

Parliamentarians are leaders in society and have both the mandate and the public confidence to act in the interests of the community and respond to the HIV crisis. Parliamentarians vote for the Budget and can command the influence and resources required to improve the national response to HIV/AIDS in their countries. As representatives of the people, parliamentarians are in a unique position to set an example, raise awareness of HIV and spur others into action.

The fight against HIV/AIDS requires strong policy-making and the development of national programmes that look beyond the health impact of HIV and address the myriad challenges created by the pandemic. Successful policies and programmes require ongoing monitoring and scrutiny to ensure proper implementation; parliamentarians must play this fundamental oversight role.

The purpose of this study is, in part, to respond directly to concerns from African parliamentarians about what various parliaments across Africa are doing about HIV/AIDS. It provides lessons learned and detailed analysis on the impact of parliamentary oversight of HIV/AIDS in a number of countries in Africa. This research also contributes key recommendations to strengthen the role of parliamentarians in the fight against HIV/AIDS. Whether it be the enactment of laws to prohibit discrimination against People Living With HIV/AIDS (PLWHAs) or budgetary oversight to ensure HIV programmes receive adequate funding, the full engagement of parliamentarians is critical to ensure effective national responses to the pandemic and adequate resources to support such initiatives.

In recognition of the crucial role of parliamentarians in the fight against HIV/AIDS, and because of the growing field of inquiry which has recently opened to look at the governance challenges in combating the spread of HIV/AIDS in Africa, the Canadian PC approached IDASA to undertake research on the practice of oversight in various African parliaments with respect to HIV/AIDS. This publication is the product of a growing partnership between the Parliamentary Centre and IDASA, who share a commitment to the promotion of good governance and improved accountability of policy-makers.

We hope that parliamentarians and other actors in the field of governance will be able to make use of this research in advancing the response to HIV/AIDS within their countries and at a regional and international level.

Christine Ivory, Regional Coordinator, Parliamentary Support Programme
Dr. Rasheed Draman, Director, Africa Programmes
Dr. Steven Langdon, Director, Africa-Canada Parliamentary Support Programme

1. Introduction

1.1 Problem statement

There is sufficient consensus that HIV/AIDS presents a crisis to societies and that the multi-sectoral impact of the pandemic demands a multi-sectoral response. This means role-players from different sectors must participate both in framing the issues as well as in the responses. An analysis of the institutions and their specific interventions will indicate that there is either insufficient political responses or that the political responses have not sufficiently added to the solution.

The Governance and AIDS Programme of IDASA (IDASA-GAP) and the Canadian Parliamentary Centre (PC) investigated the role of parliamentary oversight in national HIV/AIDS responses. Parliaments have been requested to engage with HIV/AIDS from a legislative point of view. They make and review laws and policies to deal with the problems of HIV/AIDS. In addition, individual Members of Parliament (MPs) have been requested to provide leadership in their constituencies and at national level. However, the institutional mechanisms required to support individual MPs in their efforts are not described. Furthermore, the political dimensions of parliament as a democratic institution have not been sufficiently investigated.

1.2 Background

Since the first diagnosis of AIDS more than two decades ago, many aspects of the pandemic have been and continue to be the subject of intensive investigation. These include the bio-medical, social, cultural, economic and political aspects of the pandemic. This research by IDASA-GAP and the Canadian PC focuses on the effective use of parliamentary oversight in the national responses to HIV/AIDS. This specific enquiry is part of a broader theme of governance and HIV/AIDS and seeks to illustrate the need for stronger and sustained democratic governance practices to help societies manage the pandemic more effectively as well as lay the foundation for a more equal, democratic society in which HIV/AIDS is normalised and no longer a crisis.

The research is an assessment of how the national parliaments of Botswana, Ghana, Kenya, Mozambique and South Africa use their oversight function to inform and monitor the national HIV/AIDS responses. Participating, and where applicable, other African parliaments can use the findings and recommendations to improve the oversight function in their HIV/AIDS responses.

On completion of the baseline study, there were two dissemination processes of the preliminary findings, providing opportunities for MPs to consider and comment on these findings and share their experiences in relation to the themes reflected in the recommendations. In September 2005 the Canadian PC convened a Policy Dialogue Forum in Senegal[1] where the preliminary findings were presented. In February 2006 IDASA-GAP and the Canadian PC convened a Regional Policy Dialogue Forum in South Africa. At this latter meeting MPs had an opportunity to reflect not only on the findings but also to design practical interventions in light of the recommendations.[2]

This research and the dissemination of its findings are part of a broader strategy by the Canadian PC and IDASA-GAP to build a critical mass of MPs who will play a prominent role in the analysis, framing and evaluation of the national responses to HIV/AIDS.

1.3   Rationale for the research

The primary goal of the research was to identify ways to improve the overall effectiveness of the HIV/AIDS responses in the participating countries. A complex set of cultural, social, economic and political factors converge to create an environment where people are both vulnerable and susceptible to HIV/AIDS. As a result, researchers and AIDS activists advocate for a multi-sectoral response so as to harness optimal resources (including human, financial and infrastructure) and expertise.

While a multi-sectoral approach attempts to be as inclusive as possible of government, non-government and civil society institutions, parliaments are conspicuously absent. Yet, this research illustrates that parliaments, as representative institutions with law-making and oversight functions as their core business, can make a positive contribution to the effectiveness of the HIV/AIDS response.

Government leads the response to HIV/AIDS. In all of the participating countries, the Executive informs the process of analysis of the pandemic, guides the development of the responses and monitors those responses. In many instances, non-state actors assist government in implementing the responses, but government remains the lead agency. On the other hand, parliaments have a moral and legal authority to monitor government business. This is part of their core business within the democratic governance framework.

Parliaments should therefore play a central role in assessing the status quo and the impact of HIV/AIDS and influencing the responses. This makes HIV/AIDS one of the thematic areas for the application of the more objective functions of parliaments, i.e. law-making and oversight. Parliaments can ensure that HIV/AIDS remain a priority agenda item on the government business programmes and that all government sectors are involved in the implementation and monitoring of their respective programmatic and budgetary responses.

The assertion is that the considered and effective involvement of parliament in the pandemic translates into a more effective response to HIV/AIDS and therefore adds value to the maintenance of democracy, resulting in a society able to cope much better with the impact of the pandemic.

Placing any limitation on the role of parliaments in determining HIV/AIDS priorities undermines an effective response to HIV/AIDS and undermines the power of democratic governance. The weakened democracy may then continue to be a feature of the post-AIDS society.

In spite of the importance of parliaments in ensuring good democratic practice, researchers from all the participating countries had difficulty finding a significant body of literature describing the role of parliaments in determining HIV/AIDS priorities. This was particularly the case in relation to parliamentary oversight. At the same time they could find an overwhelming number of studies and texts on the role of the Executive with regard to HIV/AIDS. This includes information on interventions by the offices of heads of states (Presidents, Prime Ministers or their deputies, depending on the title within different countries), Departments of Health and to some extent other government departments.

They also found insufficient information on the challenges facing parliaments to guide the institutions' engagement in HIV/AIDS-related issues. These constraints informed the rationale for the study and the framing of the research questions.

The study objectives, conclusions and recommendations are squarely placed within these constraints. Recommendations aim to take these conditions into account, recognising that there is an ideal to strive towards but, while doing so, carving out a democratic space by parliaments is an ongoing process. This research is an attempt to assist and facilitate that process.

2. Parliaments, politics and HIV – the research project

2.1 Objectives of the study

The overall objective of the research project was to determine whether parliaments can and have made significant contributions to the national HIV/AIDS responses, in particular via the use of the parliamentary oversight function. The research sought to:

- Generate information and, where possible, new knowledge that will assist in increasing the effectiveness of the HIV/AIDS responses;
- Clarify the roles and responsibilities of parliaments in the context of the multi-sectoral responses to HIV/AIDS;
- Understand and apply the parliamentary oversight function in an innovative manner within the complex environment of HIV/AIDS.

2.2 Methodology

The study was primarily a desk/literature review supplemented by key informant interviews. In respect of the literature review, the main data sources were secondary data, including Hansard and other publications on parliamentary proceedings such as those produced by the Parliamentary Monitoring Group (in South Africa) as well as academic and media publications.

Key informant interviews were conducted to test some of the information gathered in the desk review. Interviewees included MPs and, in certain countries, officials from National AIDS Authorities (NAAs), government departments and ministries, and selected civil society organisations (CSOs).

2.3   Selecting the countries

Botswana, Ghana, Kenya, Mozambique and South Africa participated in the project. A number of considerations influenced the choice of countries. One was the regional spread; another was current activities of either IDASA-GAP or the Canadian PC in the countries which facilitated access to researchers, research institutions and key informant interviewees. A third consideration was differences in electoral systems: three countries (Botswana, Ghana, Kenya) follow a first-past-the-post (FPTP) electoral system and the other two countries (Mozambique and South Africa) have a list-proportional (PR) system. This provides an opportunity for assessing how parliamentary oversight functions in different electoral systems. Varying HIV prevalence rates was another consideration. Ghana has the lowest, at 3–4% nationally, and Botswana the highest at about 36%. This allows a comparison between countries where the pandemic is not a high priority issue and countries where it has been declared an emergency by government.

2.4   The research questions

To facilitate the collection of data and the overall conceptualisation of the project, the following research questions were formulated.

1. HIV, AIDS and parliamentary systems: Are parliaments able to maintain their institutional capacity – as a workplace and a legislative body – in order to exercise oversight effectively?
2. HIV, AIDS and the electoral system: How can electoral systems provide for effective and legitimate representation in order to ensure effective oversight?
3. Oversight by parliamentary committees: Which parliamentary committees are focusing on HIV/AIDS and what are the specific HIV/AIDS-related issues which these committees focus on?
4. Parliamentary committees and the political leadership: What is the nature of the interaction, if any, between the parliamentary committees and the offices of the head of state as well as the health ministries?
5. Parliamentary committees and extra-parliamentary institutions: What is the nature of the interaction between the parliamentary committees and the NAAs as well as the Auditor-Generals' offices?
6. Public participation: To what extent do citizens participate in the parliamentary oversight process and how is this done?
7. Legislative protection of PLWHAs: What mechanisms have parliaments adopted in respect of the influx of generic drugs and distribution of antiretroviral therapy (ART)? How have parliaments dealt with the criminalisation of wilful transmission of HIV?
8. MPs as AIDS advocates: Are MPs able to act as AIDS advocates in parliament and in their constituencies?

2.5   Research challenges

The use of case studies

This research is time-bound and serves a snap shot of the involvement of five national parliaments in their respective national responses to HIV/AIDS. This particular kind of methodology presents advantages and disadvantages. One particular advantage is it provides an opportunity for a detailed assessment of particular HIV/AIDS-related issues as they are manifest at a particular time and place, governed by certain specific conditions at that particular time. It enables one to zoom in on particular issues providing a set of recommendations specific to geographic location and time. In addition, one is able to compare different scenarios at a particular point in time.

However, to track the progress of each of these national situations one would have to conduct later studies to evaluate follow-up to recommendations and lessons learnt. This could either require re-visiting the same institutions and countries at a future date or doing the same study with similar institutions in different countries.

For both IDASA-GAP and the Canadian PC, the case study methodology proved the best option as it informs future activities based on the research findings in the participating countries.

The research budget

All researchers reported the limited budget as a barrier to covering all the issues in their terms of reference and at the depth they were requested to. This resulted in, for example, limiting the number of key informant interviews and restricting the investigation into oversight activities to parliamentary/House-based ones.

Access to MPs and parliamentary resource people and information

This was certainly one of the most common obstacles facing researchers. The main reasons for lack of access to MPs for interviews were that the research coincided with parliamentary elections, busy schedules or bureaucratic procedures.

Further, in some countries research into legislative oversight of HIV/AIDS had never been conducted before which meant that MPs and other key informant interviewees had to familiarise themselves with the concepts before being able to respond to the specific issues.

In general however it should be noted that there was no compromise on the actual research project and the data reported. The only obvious drawback was a considerable narrowing of the research brief and terms of reference.

3. The significance of parliamentary oversight

3.1 Defining parliamentary oversight

Parliamentary oversight can be considered as part of the role of parliaments to 'share, in varying respects, the function of providing some form of link between the government and the governed.'[3] MPs give voice to the aspirations of the people.

Parliament uses its internal mechanisms and processes to act as an interface between government and the people – this is essentially the nature of representative democracy. A parliament that takes up this role in a serious and consistent manner will conceive of the oversight function as being accountable to the people, i.e. citizens and non-citizens, voters and those who may be barred from voting because of age or immigrant status. All people, regardless of their status as eligible voters, are vulnerable and susceptible to HIV/AIDS.

When parliamentary oversight is understood in a broader context, its practice is able to contribute to the achievement of the democratic principles of transparent and accountable government. In the process of exercising oversight, parliament monitors the nature and extent of the exercise of executive authority, including whether the stated objectives are being met and are responsive to the needs of the people.

Parliament can only achieve a significant measure of success if it ensures both quantitative (how many of the expected results are the Executive meeting?) and qualitative (how is the Executive meeting its goals and what is the impact?) government accountability.

Therefore, parliamentary oversight cannot be restricted to a checklist of what has been done and what has not been done. Instead, it should comprise a comprehensive examination of pre-determined goals or objectives, detailed implementation plans, delivery on those plans, measuring of the extent to which those plans have been implemented and of whether the outputs achieved the stated objectives. In addition, parliamentary oversight should involve an enquiry into the overall impact of the outputs in terms of a national framework which, depending on the country, could be contained in one or more national plans. This necessitates an enquiry into the process of determining the goals, compiling the plans and other planning and programming functions.

3.2 Distinguishing between oversight and law-making

Parliamentary oversight should be distinguished from legislative functions, i.e. approving or amending laws and monitoring and evaluating the implementation of law/policy.

Illustration: Constitution of South Africa and role of parliament

The South African Constitution illustrates clearly the distinction between the legislative role of parliament and its oversight role. In Section 42(3) it states that parliament houses the representatives of the people to ensure 'government by the people under the constitution' and inter alia, that the National Assembly '...is elected to represent the people and to ensure government by the people under the Constitution. It does this by choosing the president, by providing a national forum for public consideration of issues, by passing legislation and by scrutinising and overseeing Executive action.'[4]

At least two other sections expand on and enhance one's understanding of section 42(3). These are sections 55(2) and 56. Firstly, section 55(2) grants express authority to parliament to 'hold organs of state in the national sphere accountable, and to exercise oversight over national Executive authority and organs of the state'. This sub-section thus empowers the National Assembly to 'provide for mechanisms (a) to ensure that all executive organs of state in the national sphere of government are accountable to it; and (b) to maintain oversight of (i) the exercise of national executive authority, including the implementation of legislation; and (ii) any organ of state'.

Secondly, section 56 describes the minimum standards of accountability for the exercise of the above-mentioned oversight. The National Assembly 'or any of its committees may (a) summon any person to appear before it to give evidence on oath or affirmation, or to produce documents; (b) require any person or institution to report to it; (c) compel, in terms of national legislation or the rules and orders, any person or institution to comply with a summons or requirement in terms of paragraph (a) or (b); and receive petitions, representations or submissions from any interested persons or institutions'.

In addition to the above, the National Assembly must '(a) facilitate public involvement in the legislative and other processes of the Assembly and its committees; and (b) conduct its business in an open manner, and hold its sittings, and those of its committees, in public, but reasonable measures may be taken (i) to regulate public access, including access of the media, to the Assembly and its committees; and (ii) to provide for the searching of any person and, where appropriate, the refusal of entry to, or the removal of, any person. The National Assembly may not exclude the public, including the media, from a sitting of a committee unless it is reasonable and justifiable to do so in an open and democratic society'.

3.3 Parliamentary mechanisms and institutions for oversight

The oversight function can be implemented in several different ways. House-based, or internal, oversight occurs while parliament is in session and this is normally via the assembly or parliamentary committees.

Assembly-based oversight

While there are a number of mechanisms available to MPs while meeting as the assembly, the one cited in this report is parliamentary questions. The rules of parliament provide for MPs to address questions to ministers or the head of state related to any public matter that falls within the official portfolio of the respective ministers or within the responsibilities of the head of state. Questions may be used to elicit information or to request government action on a certain matter.

Parliamentary committees

Without exception, all parliaments constitute smaller working groups, referred to as parliamentary committees, in which much of the in-depth work of parliament is carried out. As stated above, the focus of this research is on committees shadowing specific government departments or ministries known either as Select, Portfolio or Working Committees.

The number of committees in each parliament is predominantly influenced by two factors, i.e. the oversight focus areas (for example, health, transport, education, trade, etc.) and the number of MPs. The core functions of these committees are to monitor the work of the respective department, contribute to or participate in debates, amend bills and organise public hearings if an issue is of great public interest. Committees may also initiate bills. In the course of their oversight work, committees may summon any person to give evidence or to produce documents, and they can require any person or institution to report to them.

The committee's brief is broad enough for it to work on a particular focus area allocated to it, e.g. health or finance. This includes the authority to:
- Monitor and oversee the work of national government departments, including overseeing the department's finances and holding them accountable;
- Oversee the accounts of state institutions;
- Examine specific areas of public life or matters of public interest and organise public hearings on such matters;
- Initiate, consider or debate bills and amend them;
- Consider private members' and provincial legislative proposals and special petitions;
- Summon anyone to give evidence or produce documents before the committee;
- Require any person or institution to report to the committee;
- Consider international treaties and agreements;
- Take care of domestic parliamentary issues.

The benefits of parliamentary committees include:[5]
- Increasing the amount of work that can be done – it is more efficient for a large group to delegate its work to smaller groups than to try to do it all in a single group;
- Ensuring that issues can be debated in more depth than can be done in plenary sessions (because more time is available to concentrate on details);

- Increasing the participation of MPs in discussions (members of a group can participate more fully when the group is small);
- Enabling MPs to develop expertise and in-depth knowledge of the committee's area of work;
- Providing a forum for the public to present its views directly to MPs, something which is not possible in a plenary sitting of the national assembly.

The structure or content of the above forms of oversight, in particular for committee work, include:

- Key performance indicators and departmental strategic plans;
- Annual and quarterly progress reports;
- The appearance of departmental officials before committees to answer questions;
- Annual budget hearings and reviews of departmental expenditure activities using the Auditor-General's reports.

Public hearings

Members of the public, including representatives from CSOs, participate in the parliamentary process via the committees either as observers at committee meetings or through written and/or oral representations at public hearings convened by parliamentary committees.

Fieldwork-based oversight activities

These oversight activities take place when groups of MPs leave the House and visit constituencies and institutions (such as schools or clinics) or particular government programmes (such as feeding schemes, land reform programmes or training programmes).

While House-based, as opposed to fieldwork-based, oversight activities are more cost-effective, they have a number of limitations. These include denying MPs information from primary sources, i.e. the recipients of government services. They also limit the extent of interaction between MPs and constituencies or the people they represent. This is particularly important in the context of a proportional electoral system where MPs are elected according to a party list and not directly by constituencies. Another limitation, linked to the first two, is that MPs are reliant on information from government departments and selected private and civil society sector representatives. Essentially, usually only institutions and citizens from the town or city where parliament is located have an opportunity to access MPs and parliament. This dependence on government departments and selected civil society and public sector role-players has the potential to undermine parliament's autonomy and its ability to exercise its oversight function effectively.

3.4   Oversight by other political institutions

Auditor-General

The Auditor-General's office exists within all government institutions and its role in parliamentary oversight is as an extra-parliamentary body with oversight powers over expenditure and financial systems. It aims to provide independent and objective quality audits and related value-added services in the management of public resources, thereby enhancing good governance in the public sector. The AG achieves this aim by '…conducting audits of government departments and other public sector bodies in order to provide assurance to parliament that accountable entities have achieved their financial objectives and managed their financial affairs according to sound financial principles and in accordance with the legal framework created by parliament'.[6]

One critical parliamentary committee that works with the Auditor-General is the Parliamentary Accounts Committee (PAC) which is tasked with examining the Auditor-General's reports to determine whether spending by government departments complies with the legislature's intentions and expected standards, and whether value for money is obtained.

Opposition/minority parties

Opposition MPs play a very important role in parliamentary oversight. Firstly, the minority leader is the principal spokesperson for the minority representation within parliament. Secondly, the main function of minority party MPs within parliament involves challenging the ruling party on issues relating to the socio-economic conditions of the country as well as red flag concerns of public interest. To play this role, opposition members may ask questions during portfolio committee meetings, or may submit questions to any senior government official for oral answers in plenary sessions of the assembly.

4. HIV, AIDS and democratic challenges

All of the countries included in the study faced enormous challenges in the establishment and maintenance of democratic governance even before HIV/AIDS became a crisis within those societies.

Botswana

In 1965, Botswana gained independence from Britain. It is one of the most stable countries in the region as it has had the longest run of peaceful political activity and is one of the richest. From a democratic governance perspective therefore, it should be the one with the most stable environment that nurtures democracy. The Executive is very dominant in the response to HIV/AIDS with the President's involvement hailed as positive in many sectors in and outside of Botswana. This poses a particular challenge to the Botswana Legislature as the response to HIV/AIDS has largely been devoid of any democratic processes.

Ghana

Ghana, with its universal, free and fair electoral system, was in 1957 the first colony in Africa to gain independence. Its first post-independence parliament was constituted that year. Like Mozambique, Ghana has experienced intense civil wars since independence. However, 1992 – 2004 was the most stable period in its post-independent history with the establishment of the fourth republic and elections in 1992. Prior to 1992, Ghana experienced three military coups (i.e. in 1966, 1972 and 1981) and since independence has alternated between military rule and parliamentary democracy.

Kenya

Kenya, like Botswana, has experienced a fairly stable democracy with no armed conflict following independence from Britain in 1963.

Mozambique

In 1975, Mozambique gained independence from Portugal and, as noted above, has had to deal with post-independence conflict for many years. At the end of Portuguese rule in 1975, Frelimo established a one-party state eliminating political pluralism. The-post liberation period was characterised by intense civil war and sabotage led by the rebel forces, Renamo. Only the 1990 constitutional reforms ended the state's formal commitment to a single-party state and introduced free multi-party elections and a market-based economy. A 1992 peace agreement officially ended the civil war.

South Africa

Prior to 1990, South Africa under the National Party was self-ruled and professed to be a democratic state but it only really became a democracy after the first inclusive elections in 1994. Its transition to democracy from 1990-1994 was marked by extensive political negotiations which influenced the process of drafting the first national AIDS plan. South Africa's response is characterised by highly democratic processes, particularly in the early 1990s. However, this has become politically contested terrain, which is not helpful for effective management of the pandemic.

A well-functioning democratic institution requires a well-functioning democratic society with democrats who willingly participate in the system and adhere to the rules of democracy.[7] This is not achieved overnight and seems more likely to happen in countries with a longer history of democratic practice. The overall advantage of this for HIV/AIDS is effective service delivery. For the five countries included in this study democratic experience and number of years since independence do not seem to be indicators of a stable or mature democracy. Economic, political and social upheavals severely affect the maintenance of a strong democratic governance system and all of these countries should be considered young democracies.

Generally the relatively short history of democratic governance means that the parliaments in the participating countries continue to struggle for their rightful place and to establish their authority. They are of course not assisted in their efforts by the global trend towards greater Executive power.[8]

The democratic trajectory of these countries, in particular their parliaments, should thus be brought into the equation when considering the theoretical ideal of the roles and responsibilities of parliaments in general and in particular in the context of HIV/AIDS.

5. Research findings

5.1 HIV, AIDS and parliamentary systems: Are parliaments able to maintain their institutional capacity – as a workplace and a legislative body – to exercise oversight effectively?

Data about the actual impact of HIV/AIDS on parliaments in terms of people infected and affected is not available. However, all of the country-specific reports indicate that the pandemic has had some impact on parliaments in all of the countries.

In South Africa and Kenya there is evidence that parliaments are considering HIV/AIDS from an organisational perspective, including considering the impact of the pandemic on the parliament as a workplace. These parliaments provide some form of HIV/AIDS information to MPs and support/administrative staff.

There is also evidence that Kenyan MPs face increasing demands to spend time attending to sick relatives, attending funeral rites for constituents and participating in resource mobilisation to assist those affected and infected by HIV/AIDS. The overall effect is MPs spend time on HIV/AIDS-related commitments due to illness, funerals and caring for the sick and orphaned. At an institutional level, this compromises their ability to participate effectively in parliamentary deliberations leading to delays in passing legislation. Further, nearly 60% of Kenyans live below the poverty line and therefore MPs are expected to play a leading role in harambees to mobilise funds for their constituents for funeral expenses and school fees for orphaned children.

5.2 HIV, AIDS and the electoral system: How can electoral systems provide for effective and legitimate representation to ensure effective oversight?

There is no evidence in the reports that any of the five parliaments or individual MPs consider the issues of HIV/AIDS in this manner. Strand and Chirambo (2004) begin to explore the relationship between HIV, AIDS and electoral processes and elucidate some of the linkages that should be explored by MPs.[9]

The representation of women in parliament is integral to effective oversight and equitable representation. The study found that all five parliaments include women representatives but only in Mozambique and South Africa is representation by women in parliament above 30%. Both countries follow a proportional representation (PR) system. This allows for easier accommodation of the interests of special/vulnerable groups. The 30% target for the representation of women has been agreed to by the Southern African Development Community (SADC) parliaments and is being monitored by the SADC Parliamentary Forum. This gender-based target for parliamentary representation is said to encourage the advancement of women as political leaders and recognises their contributions to effective governance.

RANK	Country	Lower/single House			
		Elections	Seats*	Women	% Women
81	Botswana	10 2004	63	7**	11.1
82	Ghana	12 2004	230	25	10.9
"	Kenya	12 2002	224	16	7.1
9	Mozambique	12 2004	250	87	34.8
13	South Africa***	4 2004	400	131	32.8

Table 1: Women representatives in parliament following 2004 elections[10]

Notes: * Figures correspond to the number of seats currently filled in parliament.
** All seven female representatives in Botswana come from the ruling party.
*** South Africa: the figures on the distribution of seats do not include the 36 special rotating delegates appointed on an ad-hoc basis, and the percentages given are therefore calculated on the basis of 54 permanent seats.

5.3 Oversight by parliamentary committees: Which parliamentary committees are focusing on HIV/AIDS and what are the specific HIV/AIDS-related issues which these committees focus on?

All five parliaments use the committee system and within different parliaments HIV/AIDS is the focus of a number of different committees. Depending on the structure of parliament, each parliament has a specific committee on HIV/AIDS oversight, the primary committee, while a number of parliaments have one or two other committees that occasionally consider the pandemic.

Table 2: Parliamentary committees and HIV/AIDS					
FUNCTION	**South Africa**	**Botswana**	**Ghana**	**Kenya**	**Mozambique**
Financial oversight	Standing Committee on Public Accounts	Public Accounts Committee/ Finance and Estimates Committee	Finance Committees	Parliamentary Accounts Committee	Planning and Finance Committee
Health sector management	Health Committee	Health Committee	Select Committee on Health	Parliamentary Committee on Health, Housing, Labour & Social Welfare	Social Affairs, Gender and Environment Committee
Primary committee that deals with issues related to HIV/AIDS	Health Committee	Special Select Committee on HIV/AIDS (ad hoc established in 1998)	Select Committee on Health	Parliamentary Committee on Health, Housing, Labour & Social Welfare	Social Affairs, Gender and Environment Committee
Parliament staff AIDS education	Office of the Secretary to Parliament: Human Resources	Parliamentary Staff Committee on HIV/AIDS		Parliamentary Committee on Health, Housing, Labour & Social Welfare	Social Affairs, Gender and Environment Committee

The internal institutional capacity and available resources directly influence the work of the individual parliamentary committees.

Institutional mechanisms: size of parliament and structure of representation

The number of seats per parliament is an important factor in effective oversight. Of the participating countries, Botswana has the smallest parliament with 63 seats and South Africa the largest with 400 MPs. In Botswana, the previous chair of the parliamentary AIDS committee served on seven committees in addition to being the party whip in parliament. In the current Botswana parliament, the biggest since independence, MPs can be a member of as many as four committees.

The Social Affairs, Gender and Environment Committee (CASGA) in the Mozambique parliament illustrates the challenges of a committee with a very broad scope. CASGA is responsible for HIV/AIDS in addition to:
- Education;
- Culture;
- Youth;
- Sports;
- Gender;
- Ensuring the protection of the family, children and the promotion of women's issues;
- Protecting and promoting the environment;

- Protecting and promoting cultural patrimony;
- Promoting employment;
- Protection of employees;
- Social security;
- Re-allocation and protection of demobilised soldiers;
- Population;
- Protection of people with disabilities;
- Religious activities.

Administrative and research support for committees and individual MPs

In Botswana, MPs confirmed that another key factor undermining their oversight role is their limited technical support and access to research facilities. Unfortunately, the requirement that committees table all research reports to parliament is not always met because of gaps in research. Some MPs reported that most of the time they do not even really know what research and information they need. It has been suggested that parliament should outsource administrative services, which would help the House tremendously. Although this is seen as a likely solution for this problem, lack of financial resources remains a major constraint.

In contrast, South Africa seems to be well-resourced compared to the other parliaments. It has an extensive pool of researchers with sectoral expertise available to committees and individual MPs. Committees also have dedicated support/administrative staff to assist committee chairpersons.

Central coordinating office within parliament

This office, sometimes referred to as the Secretary to Parliament, can inter alia help mainstream HIV/AIDS across committees. To a large extent, HIV/AIDS is presented in parliament as a health issue and mainly by MPs advocating for a particular issue such as prevention. South Africa and Kenya are the only countries where committees other than health have consistently discussed HIV/AIDS in interactions with government departments. The need to make HIV/AIDS part of the core business of all parliamentary committees is reflected in the expansive nature of the pandemic.

Oversight in the assembly and not parliamentary committees

While there is general consensus that oversight within committees is ideal, this does not however exclude important oversight work that can be done within the assembly. The Botswana assembly illustrates this. In the appendix on page 29 is a list of issues raised by MPs since 1995 indicating that MPs have been monitoring government's programme.

Basics for effective parliamentary oversight of HIV and AIDS

- Design methods that allow parliaments to work with the known, the unknown and the contradictions of HIV and AIDS;
- Design an effective framework for oversight of HIV and AIDS;
- Prioritise the issues; navigating the complex terrain of HIV and AIDS;
- Transform Budget oversight so that the Budget becomes the critical pillar for HIV and AIDS oversight;
- Share experience of democratic governance in the context of HIV and AIDS;
- Respect the separation of powers and therefore respect the legal and moral authority of parliament;
- Provide written and well-published policy or law on roles and responsibilities of parliament;
- Ensure that parliament becomes a representation of the voice of the people experiencing HIV and AIDS;
- Strengthen the representation of women and AIDS in parliament;
- Effective, well resourced and proactive parliamentary committees;
- Political leadership displayed by MPs and members of the Executive alike;
- Well-resourced, independent and vocal extra-parliamentary institutions such as the office of the Auditor-General, independent media and an engaged civil society;
- Individual MPs as advocates and role models in HIV and AIDS;
- Parliamentary focal point for HIV and AIDS – sub-committee or full parliamentary committee on HIV and AIDS or multi-party, non-partisan committee on HIV and AIDS;
- Adequate institutional support and capacity to undertake effective oversight of HIV and AIDS;
- Active and informed citizens who believe and participate in democracy;
- Legislative framework for the protection and promotion of the rights of people infected and affected by HIV and AIDS.

5.4 Parliamentary committees and the political leadership: What is the nature of the interaction, if any, between the parliamentary committees and the offices of the heads of state as well as the health ministries?

The interaction between parliaments and leaders is restricted to ministers who report on HIV/AIDS to the respective parliamentary committees. There was no evidence in any of the countries of consistent and regular interaction between the heads of state and parliamentary committees. That kind of interaction is limited to the times when the head of state addresses the assembly and refers to HIV/AIDS in his address.

5.5 Parliamentary committees and extra-parliamentary institutions: What is the nature of the interaction between the parliamentary committees and the NAAs as well as the Auditor-Generals' offices?

National AIDS Authorities

NAAs are considered part of the Executive and generally parliaments interact with them via the department and/or ministry of health. Ghana is the exception in that the Ghana AIDS Commission (GAC) Act stipulates that parliament oversees the functions of the GAC thereby providing for the Director-General of the GAC to submit reports directly to parliament. As far as the researchers were able to establish, this is the only instance where a formal and direct oversight relationship exists between an NAA and parliament.

There has, however, been interaction between the NAA and parliament or individual MPs on many other levels, though largely related to health issues. In countries where the NAA was established as a result of an act of parliament, MPs were involved in passing this law. In addition, the NAA in Kenya has also been working closely with the parliamentary Committee on Health to ensure that policy guidelines and mechanisms for disbursement and management of resources are established. It has also been interacting with individual MPs and the parliamentary Committee on Health, Housing, Labour and Social Welfare.

Ghana is the only country where there is a formal partnership between parliament and the GAC in the form of the Parliamentarians against HIV/AIDS Project. In Mozambique and South Africa one or more MPs serve on the governing structure of the NAA. In certain instances, MPs or parliamentary committees receive funding from the NAA or the latter assists in training MPs. In some countries the NAA and parliament (Health Committee MPs) conduct joint campaigns to raise awareness about HIV/AIDS and increase the level of interaction. Examples of these are in Mozambique, Kenya and Ghana.

Auditor-General

All parliaments make use of the reports by the Auditor-General mainly to monitor expenditure of funding for HIV/AIDS. The evidence indicates that there is consensus about the usefulness of reports of this nature. The effective use of this mechanism in the oversight process, however, faces a number of obstacles, including lack of capacity within the Auditor-General's office and a tangential issue of the timing of the Auditor-General's investigations and release of the reports.

5.6 Public participation: To what extent do citizens participate in the parliamentary oversight process and how is this done?

Public hearings are held on a regular basis only in South Africa. All the other parliaments have irregular contact with civil society or the public. In Ghana and Mozambique, there were public hearings only in respect of the GAC Bill and the Law 5/2002 respectively. The lack of public presence even during 'open' committee meetings was noted as a major concern in Botswana.

It should be noted that this kind of interaction obviously requires a robust, informed and well-resourced civil society because all parliaments have rules providing for public hearings even if they are not convening these. The South African experience confirms that a high level of civil society activism contributes to greater interaction between organised civil society and parliament.

5.7 Legislative protection of PLWHAs: What mechanisms have parliaments adopted in respect of the influx of generic drugs and distribution of ART? How have parliaments dealt with the criminalisation of wilful transmission of HIV?

While the legislative function was not under examination *per se* in this study, the nature and content of the legal and human rights responses to the HIV/AIDS pandemic can be indicative of the legislature's priorities. The literature revealed two critical issues: firstly, laws or policies regulating the influx of generic drugs and distribution of ARVs and secondly, the criminalisation of wilful transmission of HIV.

Concerning the latter, all parliaments have at some point since the onset of the pandemic considered legal provisions for the criminalisation of the wilful transmission of HIV. In South Africa, where there is perhaps the clearest indication of the consideration of this issue, the South African Law Commission undertook extensive research to determine ways of responding to the public calls for the use of criminal law in HIV transmission. While there is no definitive law in any country criminalising wilful HIV transmission, it has returned to the table for discussion by legislatures, in particular with calls for the regional harmonisation of laws relating to HIV/AIDS.

The issue of generic drugs and the distribution of ARVs is complex and parliaments recognise the continental and sub-regional nature of this issue. Where discussed within parliaments, the issues are confined to importing of drugs and mechanisms for local manufacturing. Distribution of ARVs is largely a policy/Executive function and parliaments intervene on this topic mainly to monitor governments' targets for roll-out of ARVs. South Africa currently has the largest ARV programme in the public health sector and the Health Committee closely monitors government's progress, even if not in an overtly critical manner.

5.8 MPs as AIDS advocates: Are MPs able to act as AIDS advocates in parliament and in their constituencies?

In all parliaments there are individual MPs who are extremely vocal about HIV/AIDS either within parliamentary committees or in the assembly. Of particular significance are the dedicated efforts by chairpersons of committees responsible for HIV/AIDS who continue to lead by example the consistent investigation of the Executive's response to the pandemic. In some of the countries, such as South Africa, opposition MPs are also taking a very active role in monitoring the AIDS response.

6. Recommendations and conclusions

6.1 HIV, AIDS and parliamentary systems: Are parliaments able to maintain their institutional capacity – as a workplace and a legislative body – to exercise oversight effectively?

Parliament is an important democratic institution and one can certainly make a case for the involvement of parliament and MPs in the response to HIV/AIDS. In that regard, it is important that parliaments consider not only the policy and legislative implications of the effect of HIV/AIDS but also the institutional implications. Although the evidence is not conclusive, it does indicate that parliaments are not taking this broader view. There seems to be an emphasis on some form of legislative response with little attention being paid to the organisational impact. Literature on the impact of HIV/AIDS on the workplace[11] (or on institutions) provides overwhelming evidence that the pandemic impacts on institutions and parliament, as a workplace, is certainly not excluded from this. A further and related issue to be considered by all parliaments is the potential loss of institutional memory. What distinguishes parliament from other workplaces is that it is a significant democratic institution and it is therefore important that parliament continues to be effective.

6.2 HIV, AIDS and the electoral system: How can electoral systems provide for effective and legitimate representation to ensure effective oversight?

This is an area that requires further investigation and, as mentioned above, the current study by IDASA-GAP on HIV/AIDS and electoral systems in five African countries will shed more light on this topic. A specific issue to be examined is identifying the most appropriate electoral system that can facilitate effective representation of citizens on issues such as HIV/AIDS by allowing for rigorous oversight of the pandemic. One of the questions in this regard is the level of representation generally, and of women specifically.

In Botswana, Mozambique and South Africa – among the SADC countries worst affected by HIV/AIDS – the ruling party enjoys an overwhelming majority representation in parliament.

At the end of the Budget year and without delay, parliament must be able to voice its opinion on the performance of the Budget through a Budget Review Mechanism. This is on the basis of a transparent, comprehensive and accurate document that outlines the Budget's performance and details the public funds involved for the year in question. This document must indicate any discrepancies between the Budget that was passed and its performance, as well as the cause of such discrepancies. The examination of the Budget would provide a crucial opportunity for evaluating the Executive's public policy.

A review process of this nature would subsequently impact on the performance, monitoring and assessment of Budget allocations for HIV/AIDS-related matters.

While this may well be a reflection of the political conditions experienced by these countries, the important issue for discussion should be how this majority representation facilitates effective oversight of HIV/AIDS. In an environment where there is consensus on the ruling party's policies, irrespective of the level of support from citizens, there may be very few opposing voices. Such situations require MPs, in particular ruling party MPs, to be more vigilant about the demands and needs of the people.

In respect of the representation of women, the literature on gender and policy-making[12] provides some insight into the fact that women representatives are generally able to bring the experiences of women to the policy debates. This is important for the legislative consideration of the HIV/AIDS issues as they pertain to women. It is therefore encouraging to note the level of representation by women[13] in the SADC parliaments. However, the critical follow-up question concerns the space available for women in these parliaments to bring that specificity to the policy-making process – it does not help to have large percentages of women represented in parliament if the policy-making process and context is predominantly patriarchal. This is certainly an issue for further investigation.

6.3 Oversight by parliamentary committees: Which parliamentary committees are focusing on HIV/AIDS and what are the specific HIV/AIDS-related issues which these committees focus on?

The research confirms that oversight of HIV/AIDS is largely confined to specific parliamentary committees, in particular those with a broad social welfare mandate. This is commendable on a number of levels. Firstly, it is an indication that parliaments have noted the seriousness of the pandemic and the need for a focus at this level. Secondly, parliament provides a special focus for HIV/AIDS within one of its specialised committees, therefore dedicating time and some of its resources to bringing the pandemic into focus on behalf of the entire parliament or assembly. Thirdly, the oversight work of the committees allows some form of public engagement as well as Executive accountability. There are three recommendations to improve oversight on the committee level:

• There needs to be more parliamentary committees that integrate HIV/AIDS into their work;
• There needs to be a more systematic framework for HIV/AIDS oversight;
• Oversight of the Budget needs to be increased and expanded.

It is commendable that each of the parliaments has institutionalised a focus on HIV/AIDS with the issue as a permanent item on the agenda of at least one parliamentary committee. There are different models for HIV/AIDS focal points in parliament: the most common is a focus on HIV/AIDS in a committee focusing on social sector aspects, i.e. health, education, etc. At various times, the committee responsible for national budgets and finance (the title differs from country to country) engages with HIV/AIDS. Another model is a formal sub-committee for HIV/AIDS, although this model may not be suitable for small parliaments such as in Botswana and Mozambique.

There is, however, a need for a more generalised, mainstreamed approach to HIV/AIDS within parliament, which requires more committees to be involved in HIV/AIDS oversight.

Internal institutional capacity: resources and staff

Larger parliaments have the obvious advantage of numbers – they have more MPs to allocate to parliamentary committees. These parliaments can thus avoid members having to serve on more than one committee or committees having to deal with an extensive range of issues. This further enhances the effectiveness of oversight.

Small parliaments with fewer MPs, such as in Botswana and Mozambique, face this challenge, with MPs serving on more than one committee and with committees having combined portfolios, i.e. one committee responsible for more than one focus area and, therefore, ministry or government department. The effects of this include:

- Limited time for committees to deal in detail with issues in any one portfolio;
- Limited number of issues per portfolio can be considered;
- Prioritisation may be influenced by factors that may be personally important to the party, the MPs or the committee chairperson.

Most parliaments included in the study operate in an environment of limited resources, which impacts particularly on the availability of internal research and administrative support to MPs and parliamentary committees. Absence of technical support weakens MPs as they have virtually no independent sources of information and they thus become dependent on the Executive as their main source of information.

Both of the above issues create a barrier to effective oversight. However, it is more difficult to address issues of size than issues of resources and skills. An effective partnership with extra-parliamentary institutions is one way to meet the second challenge. These partnerships could include CSOs with research capacity and expertise as well as HIV/AIDS service providers within civil society who are in a position to comment with authority on government programmes.

6.4 Parliamentary committees and the political leadership: What is the nature of the interaction, if any, between the parliamentary committees and the offices of the heads of state as well as the health ministries?

Leaders in government interact with parliamentary committees largely on an adhoc basis. Some officials, such as Permanent Secretaries, who are also the accounting officers responsible to parliament for Executive action, may have more contact with parliament.

There are indications that direct, high-level accountability should be the preferred form of oversight, in particular given the impact of HIV/AIDS. Greater interaction with ministers and, for example, the head of the NAAs, should be promoted.

The current practice of the head of state reporting to the assembly may be accepted tradition. However, the fact that HIV/AIDS policy is increasingly moving to the highest political office in countries implies direct intervention by the head of state in this process. This kind of active leadership and the emergency presented by HIV/AIDS demands a reconsideration of this tradition. Perhaps parliaments should consider requesting the head of state, in addition to the relevant ministers, to meet on a regular basis with the various committees responsible for HIV/AIDS.

6.5   Parliamentary committees and extra-parliamentary institutions: What is the nature of the interaction between the parliamentary committees and the NAAs as well as the Auditor-Generals' offices?

There are a number of extra-parliamentary institutions that can assist parliamentary committees as well as individual MPs in the oversight of HIV/AIDS. The NAAs and the Auditor-Generals' offices were identified in this research as examples of those supporting institutions. These institutions have specific foci, resources and policy or legislative frameworks defining their functions. The potential for these institutions to improve parliamentary oversight of HIV/AIDS is recognised and has been confirmed by the results. However, improving capacity within the Auditor-Generals' offices is critical for it to be of use to parliaments and MPs. In addition, introducing a more directly accountable relationship between parliaments and the NAAs would facilitate more direct oversight of HIV/AIDS by parliaments.

6.6   Public participation: To what extent do citizens participate in the parliamentary oversight process and how is this done?

Most parliaments fall far short on the level of participation of citizens in the parliamentary oversight process. The South African parliament shows the most consistent and active civil society participation. This may be attributed to an active civil society generally, particularly in the AIDS sector. The benefits of different forms of partnerships with civil society are not being explored effectively by parliaments. Greater public access to parliamentary proceedings, such as committee meetings as open forums, would be a step in the right direction.

This is perhaps the greatest resource for all MPs and parliaments – citizens with direct experience of HIV/AIDS as well as government policy and programmes. Engagement with citizens improves the nature of representative democracy and thus oversight of HIV/AIDS. It is imperative that all parliaments ensure effective and consistent engagement with citizens.

6.7   Legislative protection of PLWHAs: What mechanisms have parliaments adopted in respect of the influx of generic drugs and distribution of ART? How have parliaments dealt with the criminalisation of wilful transmission of HIV?

All parliaments should take a more proactive role in protecting PLWHAs. There is an extensive body of evidence on the rights-based approach to HIV/AIDS arguing against the use of criminal law in a public health crisis like HIV/AIDS. Reasons for this include: criminalisation fuels discrimination, it does not lead to effective use of resources (including resources within the criminal justice system) and, more importantly, criminal law provisions cannot prevent the spread of HIV or the management of AIDS. In spite of this, parliaments periodically entertain discussions of this topic largely as a result of public calls for the use of criminal law. It would be more effective if parliaments continue to frame their deliberations within the broader human rights framework and craft a response that is consistent with the protection and promotion of human rights.

On the specific issue of access to treatment, parliaments in all countries have remained on the periphery of this discussion and debate. This, as noted above, is more complex and requires a coordinated regional response. However, it is imperative that individual parliaments consider the access to treatment and ARVs issues at national level.

From a parliamentary committee perspective, the notable absence of committees such as justice and trade and industry in HIV/AIDS oversight is further indicative of the absence of a critical debate on these issues by parliaments.

6.8   MPs as AIDS advocates: Are MPs able to act as AIDS advocates in parliament and in their constituencies?

The voices of individual MPs in the response to HIV/AIDS are becoming louder, bringing to the pandemic experiences of ordinary citizens and their engagement with HIV/AIDS. This may, at national level, be the beginnings of a movement for citizens' collective engagement with government's responses to HIV/AIDS and should be used more effectively by civil society and advocacy institutions.

Within constituencies, the issues are a lot more difficult to manage with MPs having to respond to the political priorities of the electorate. Therefore, depending on how issues are framed, the nature and extent of the responses by MPs may vary. The onerous burden is already notable in Kenya with extensive demands on the time and financial resources of MPs. What is required is a coordinated institutional response that could assist MPs in managing their responses to HIV/AIDS at local constituency level.

6.9 Other recommendations and conclusions

Expanding the response to HIV/AIDS within parliament

Currently the focus on HIV/AIDS in parliament is largely located at two levels. The first is with individuals who have a personal commitment to addressing the pandemic. A second level is with parliamentary committees that have a social welfare agenda, such as health, education and social development committees, and specific interest groups, such as women and children. Other parliamentary committees take on HIV/AIDS as and when required.

This dominance of the health and the social sector has advantages in that it brings expertise from the sector that initiated the response to HIV/AIDS. However, the disadvantage is that it prevents other role-players from contributing, which could result in obvious gaps in the response. What is lacking is a broader developmental response which, for one, will demand a multi-sectoral response to HIV/AIDS within parliament.

Increasing and expanding oversight in the Budget process

The need to increase and expand parliament's involvement in the Budget process is not a new issue and certainly not restricted to HIV/AIDS.[14] The national Budget is crucial to the successful implementation of all public projects. It combines that which is desirable, (i.e. the ambitions of an effective policy) with that which is sustainable (notably financial means). Consequently, this combination enables the Executive to strike a balance between economics and finances in its policy.

In the context of HIV/AIDS, the Budget can be used to ensure that policies that would mitigate the spread of HIV as well as enhance the living conditions of PLWHAs can be identified.

All of the parliaments play a limited role in Budget preparation as this has become more and more a policy function resting within government departments. In general, parliaments are presented with budgets already compiled, and line items and totals identified and allocated. MPs within various parliamentary committees are then required to approve these budgets. MPs can increase their role in the Budget process in the following ways:

- Ensure that budget allocations are in line with approved government priorities for HIV/ AIDS;
- Ensure that Budgets reflect additional priorities that emerge from constituency work;
- Ongoing monitoring by parliamentary committees throughout the year to ensure that government agencies are spending allocations as per approved budgets;
- Prompt annual budget reviews.

Legal or policy statements on the roles and functions of parliament

There is no doubt that parliament is an important democratic institution, with or without HIV/ AIDS, even if only in its theoretical exposition of representative democracy. The challenge is in implementing the principle of the separation of powers to ensure good governance for a vibrant and sustainable democracy.

As noted before, parliament's two core functions are firstly to make laws and policies and secondly to hold the Executive accountable. These functions have become institutionalised within the tradition of parliamentary democracy. In most countries they are also codified in constitutions and rules of parliament. The only exception to this in this study was Botswana.

The Botswana case raises different scenarios for when there is no clear framework for oversight roles and responsibilities. Firstly, it is difficult to change a tradition of exercising authority when there is no clear policy document that prescribes the authority of parliament.

Secondly, there may be a benefit in having this lacuna in the law because it allows parliament to strengthen its oversight role by pushing the boundaries imposed by the Executive. It is able to do so much more than parliaments with a detailed description of roles and functions. It does not seem that the Botswana parliament has made use of this opportunity.

Thirdly, the very detailed description of the functions of parliament, as illustrated by South Africa, is not only of benefit to parliament but could also be used by extra-parliamentary institutions as a lobbying tool to make sure that parliament performs its stipulated functions.

An attempt to become more independent

From an operational perspective, the Executive interacts with parliament as if it is attached to the office of the President, like some form of minor government department. In 1988 the Botswana parliament passed a motion urging government to take steps forthwith to ensure that parliament as a supreme body in Botswana becomes an independent institution, detached from the President's office.

Not much was done to implement this motion until 2002 when the then Speaker of parliament appointed a task force to draft terms of reference for a consultancy to assist parliament in acting on the 1988 motion. The report produced by the consultants was debated and that was all that was achieved – a debate.

Parliament adjourned without acting on the report and the matter has yet to be brought before the current parliament.

Impact on the institution

There is no or very little indication that parliaments are considering the impact of HIV/AIDS on itself as an institution in spite of the fact that all five parliaments recognise and agree with the Executive that it is an important national issue requiring political leadership. The potential impact of the pandemic on the electoral systems is one example of an issue that requires further investigation.

Representing women's voices

As noted, only two countries have more than 30% representation of women in parliament. The low levels of representation by women entrenches a largely patriarchal framework for parliamentary oversight of HIV/AIDS and silences the gender issues that should be central to this function.

It appears to be both a tragedy and an opportunity that the story of HIV/AIDS so clearly exposes continued gender inequalities in political, economic, cultural and social conditions that make women more vulnerable and susceptible to the virus. Yet the oversight function seems ill-equipped to address the pandemic in this context.

Acronyms and abbreviations

ADB	African Development Bank
AIDS	Acquired Immune Deficiency Syndrome
AMOPROC	Associacao Mocambicana para Promocao da Cidadania (Mozambican Association for the Promotion of Citizenship)
ART	Antiretroviral therapy
ARVs	Antiretrovirals
BCP	Botswana Congress Party
BDP	Botswana Democratic Party
BNF	Botswana National Front
CASGA	Comissao dos Assuntos Sociais, do Genero e Ambiente (Committee for Social Affairs, Gender and Environment), Mozambique
CBOs	Community-Based Organisations
CCG	Christian Council of Ghana
CDD	Centre for Democratic Development, Ghana
CNCS	Conselho Nacional de Combate ao SIDA (National AIDS Council), Mozambique
CNCSP	National AIDS Control Programme (Ministry of Health), Mozambique
CPP	Convention People's Party, Ghana
CSOs	Civil Society Organisations
DACF	District Assembly Common Fund, Ghana
FIDA	Federation of Women Lawyers, Ghana
FRELIMO	Frente de Libertacao de Mocambique (Mozambique's Liberation Movement)
GAC	Ghana AIDS Commission
GAP	Governance and AIDS Programme (in IDASA)
GARFUND	Ghana AIDS Response Fund
GASDE-UEM	Grupo de Activistas ANTI-SIDA e DTS- Universidade Eduardo Mondlane (Group of anti-AIDS and STDs' Activists at Eduardo Mondlane University)
GoM	Government of Mozambique
GPC	Ghana Pentecostal Council
GRNA	Ghana Registered Nurses Association
GPRS	Ghana Poverty Reduction Strategy
HIV	Human Immuno-deficiency Virus
IDASA	Institute for Democracy in South Africa
IMF	International Monetary Fund
INE	Instituto Nacional de Estatística (National Institute of Statistics), Mozambique
IPU	Inter-Parliamentary Union
JSS	Junior Secondary School
KINDLIMUKA	Associacao das Pessoas
M&E	Monitoring and Evaluation
MDA	Ministries, Departments and Agencies

MFDP	Ministry of Finance and Development Planning, Botswana
MISAU	Ministry of Health, Mozambique
MONASO	Mozambique Network of AIDS Service Organisations
MPs	Members of Parliament
NAAs	National AIDS Authorities
NACA	National AIDS Coordinating Agency, Botswana
NACP	National AIDS Control Programme, Ghana
NDC	National Democratic Congress, Ghana
NDI	National Democratic Institute
NGOs	Non-governmental organisations
NHDR	National Human Development Report
NPP	New Patriotic Party, Ghana
NUGS	National Union of Ghanaian Students
OHCS	Office of the Head of Civil Service
OTM	Organizacao dos Trabalhadores Mocambicanos (Mozambican Workers Organisation)
OVC	Orphans and Vulnerable Children
PC	Parliamentary Centre (Canadian partner on this project)
PEN	Plano Estratégico Nacional (Mozambique's National Strategic Plan for HIV/AIDS)
PLWHAs	People Living With HIV/AIDS
PMTCT	Prevention of Mother-to-Child-Transmission
PNC	People's National Convention, Ghana
PPAG	Planned Parenthood Association of Ghana
PTCT	Parent-to-Child-Transmission (of HIV)
RENAMO	Resistencia Nacional de Mocambique (Mozambique's National Resistance Movement)
SADC	Southern African Development Community
PF	Parliamentary Forum
SSS	Senior Secondary School
START	Support Treatment and Anti-Retroviral Therapy
STIs	Sexually Transmitted Infections
UN	United Nations

Endnotes

1 Presentation by Mary Caesar-Katsenga, available on www.idasa.org and see also www.parlcent.ca for information about the Policy Dialogue Forum.

2 See www.idasa.org and www.parlcent.ca for the workshop report and information on the establishment of the first Pan African Coalition of African MPs against HIV/AIDS (CAPAH).

3 Ball, A. 1993. *Modern Politics and Government*. London, MacMillan Press Ltd (Mozambique Report).

4 Constitution of the Republic of South Africa, Act 108 of 1996 (as amended).

5 http://www.parliament.gov.za/pls/portal/web_app.new_middle_column?p_page_name=PARLIAMENTARY_COMMITTEES

6 www.agsa.co.za

7 Chirambo K and M Caesar. 2003. "AIDS and Governance in Southern Africa: Emerging Theories and Perspectives". A Report on the IDASA/UNDP Regional Governance and AIDS Forum.

8 Omano, E. 2005. "A democratic developmental state in Africa? A concept paper", Centre for Policy Studies at www.cps.org.za

9 Strand P. and Chirambo K. (eds). 2005. *HIV/AIDS and Democratic Governance in South Africa: Illustrating the Impact on Electoral Processes*, IDASA. Cape Town. Also available on www.idasa.org. A further publication on this topic, but looking at Malawi, Zambia, Namibia, Botswana, Tanzania and Senegal, is due for publication in 2006.

10 www.ipu.org/wmn-e/world.htm

11 www.heard.org.za and www.cadre.org.za

12 www.genderlinks.co.za

13 www.sadcpf.org and www.genderlinks.co.za

14 See IDASA's Budget Information Service, in particular publications by the AIDS Budget Unit, on www.idasa.org

References

Kioko , U. (forthcoming) *Parliament, Politics and AIDS: The case of Kenya*. Cape Town: Idasa-GAP

Machel, J. (forthcoming) *Parliament, Politics and AIDS: The case of Mozambique*. Cape Town: Idasa-GAP

Ndlovu, N and Caesar-Katsenga, M. (forthcoming) *Parliament, Politics and AIDS: The case of South Africa*. Cape Town: Idasa-GAP

Odoro, F. (forthcoming) *Parliament, Politics and AIDS: The case of Ghana*. Cape Town: Idasa-GAP

Somolekae, G. (forthcoming) *Parliament, Politics and AIDS: The case of Botswana*. Cape Town: Idasa-GAP

Appendix: Botswana – Questions and motions on HIV/AIDS, 1995-2005	
Year of question	**Content of question (summarised)**
1995 March	Have traditional doctors also benefited from workshops on HIV?
1995 March	Should we consider keeping HIV-positive people in separate buildings because of the congestion in hospitals?
1995 March	Will the minister inform the House on the plans in place to alleviate the shortage of nursing personnel in hospitals and clinics?
1995 November	Will the minister inform the House about the efforts being made to source antiretrovirals (ARVs) to people living with HIV?
1995 December	Will the minister brief the House on bed occupancy rates by patients with AIDS-related ailments, and indicate whether the situation is worsening?
1996 February	Will the minister explain the delay in initiating a pilot home-based care model in Mole-polole and Tutume and explain how it will work?
1996 November	Will the minister explain whether it's not advisable to show AIDS films across the country so that people can see that there is AIDS?
1997 July	Is the minister aware of allegations that some doctors are selling AIDS tablets, and it is therefore necessary to give advice to the public?
1997 August	Will the minister brief parliament on research findings on AIDS in Botswana with particular reference to type and severity of virus, comparison with other countries, and recommended treatment for Botswana?
1998 March	Have there been any cases of home-based caregivers contracting HIV from their patients, and when will a clear package for the support of those giving care to AIDS orphans be put in place?
1999 June	What special measures exist to prevent the spread of HIV in major projects such as the North South Water Carrier Project, given the fact that the projects attract many people, including foreigners?
2000 February	Will the minister state the number of home-based care programme volunteers?
2000 July	Are traditional midwives included in the home-based care programme?
2000 July	What steps is government taking to negotiate with drug companies for a reduction in the price of AIDS drugs?
2001 February	Whether and what progress has been made in negotiating with drug companies on a reduction in the prices of AIDS drugs?
2001 December	When will the minister start a vigorous promotion for the use of the female condom?
2002 November	Will the minister inform parliament how many Botswana have benefited from ARV therapy to date, and state when the same therapy will be rolled out to other areas not yet covered?
2003 February	Will the minister explain the constraints faced so far in rolling out ARV therapy to all areas of the country given the enormous pressure to deliver on this programme and ensure that patients suffer the least inconvenience in accessing these drugs?
2003 February	Will the minister state what measures are in place to assist patients who are in areas surrounding major villages and towns, taking into account the fact that some patients are poor and cannot afford transport to facilities in major centres?

www.ingramcontent.com/pod-product-compliance
Lightning Source LLC
Chambersburg PA
CBHW050615290326
41929CB00063B/2919